# A Year of
# SUNDAYS

## 52 Faith & Fitness Devotions

**MARSHA APSLEY**

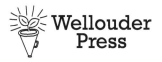

Copyright © 2021 Marsha Apsley

All rights reserved. No part of this publication may be reproduced, distributed, or transmitted in any form or by any means, including photocopying, recording, or other electronic or mechanical methods, without the prior written permission of the publisher, except in the case of brief quotations embodied in critical reviews. For permission requests, write to the author, addressed "Attention: Permissions" at marsha@marshaapsley.com

Editing support provided by Teresa Clark of The Wordsmith VA.

Cover photo by Grace Dile Photography

Scripture taken from the New King James Version®. Copyright © 1982 by Thomas Nelson. Used by permission. All rights reserved.

Scripture quotations taken from the Amplified® Bible (AMP), Copyright © 2015 by The Lockman Foundation. Used by permission. www.lockman.org

The Living Bible copyright © 1971 by Tyndale House Foundation. Used by permission of Tyndale House Publishers Inc., Carol Stream, Illinois 60188. All rights reserved. The Living Bible, TLB, and the The Living Bible logo are registered trademarks of Tyndale House Publishers.

THE HOLY BIBLE, NEW INTERNATIONAL VERSION®, NIV® Copyright © 1973, 1978, 1984, 2011 by Biblica, Inc.® Used by permission. All rights reserved worldwide. These Scriptures are copyrighted by the Biblica, Inc.® and have been made available on the Internet for your personal use only. Any other use including, but not limited to, copying or reposting on the Internet is prohibited. These Scriptures may not be altered or modified in any form and must remain in their original context. These Scriptures may not be sold or otherwise offered for sale. These Scriptures are not shareware and may not be duplicated.

Scripture quotations marked NLT are taken from the Holy Bible, New Living Translation, copyright © 1996, 2004, 2015 by Tyndale House Foundation. Used by permission of Tyndale House Publishers, Inc., Carol Stream, Illinois 60188. All rights reserved.

Scripture quotations taken from the (NASB®) New American Standard Bible®, Copyright © 1960, 1971, 1977, 1995, 2020 by The Lockman Foundation. Used by permission. All rights reserved. www.lockman.org

Published by Wellouder Press

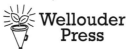

wellouderpress.com

ISBN: 978-1-7372276-4-9

# Dedication

For the women in my Faith and Fitness Membership Community — past members, present members, and members yet to come. You lovely ladies remind me to keep the main thing the main thing, and that is to keep our eyes on Jesus. We cannot pursue a healthy life before building a firm foundation of faith. Thank you for supporting this project, for offering feedback and suggestions, and for making me a better person.

# Table of Contents

Acknowledgements — xi
Introduction — xiii
Week 1 — 1
Week 2 — 5
Week 3 — 9
Week 4 — 13
Week 5 — 17
Week 6 — 21
Week 7 — 25
Week 8 — 29
Week 9 — 33
Week 10 — 37
Week 11 — 41
Week 12 — 45
Week 13 — 49
Week 14 — 53
Week 15 — 57
Week 16 — 61
Week 17 — 65
Week 18 — 69
Week 19 — 73
Week 20 — 77
Week 21 — 81
Week 22 — 85

Week 23 — 89
Week 24 — 93
Week 25 — 97
Week 26 — 101
Week 27 — 105
Week 28 — 109
Week 29 — 113
Week 30 — 117
Week 31 — 121
Week 32 — 125
Week 33 — 129
Week 34 — 133
Week 35 — 137
Week 36 — 141
Week 37 — 145
Week 38 — 149
Week 39 — 153
Week 40 — 157
Week 41 — 161
Week 42 — 165
Week 43 — 169
Week 44 — 173
Week 45 — 177
Week 46 — 181
Week 47 — 185
Week 48 — 189
Week 49 — 193
Week 50 — 197
Week 51 — 201

Week 52 — 205
Final Day — 209
Epilogue — 213

# Acknowledgements

Thanks to my running buddy Lynn who, in the early stages of this devotional, suggested this project when she had no idea I was already working on it. This was just the confirmation I needed to move forward.

Thanks to Glenneth Reed who motivates me to keep my website current. She's the reason I started posting my weekly devotions to my blog. Because of this, I realized I had content that was ready to go into another book.

A special thank you to Dr. Beth Brombosz. Without her, I would have never published my first book. Yet again, she has helped me share with you a book that I am very proud of because of all the special touches she added to it.

# Introduction

You and I are fearfully and wonderfully made. We read that in Psalm 139, but we don't always look in the mirror and see a woman like that.

I'm here to help you embrace that truth and to find freedom in living a fit and healthy life. We'll do that together by learning to honor God by honoring our bodies.

It is no accident that you have picked up this book. Get ready for a transformation, but don't worry about taking a before photo. The transformation is going to start on the inside. The outside will follow.

*A Year of Sundays* is a compilation of weekly devotions I've written since I published my first book *40 Days of Faith and Fitness*. Each devotion includes an action step. This will be your focus for the week. Meditate on the verse throughout the week and take the suggested action. When you do this, you will build your fitness on a firm foundation of faith. The result will be you living a healthy life that is sustainable.

This devotional was written to take you through an entire year. There is one entry per week followed by a suggested action step. You can use the extra space to journal your progress each week, write out a prayer, or simply reflect on God's work in your life.

Let each verse penetrate your heart and drive you to act, change your thinking, or draw you closer to the Lord.

It's time for you to start living fit and free!

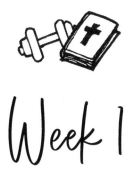

# Week 1

*For this reason we also thank God without ceasing, because when you received the word of God which you heard from us, you welcomed it not as the word of men, but as it is in truth, the word of God, which also effectively works in you who believe.*

**1 Thessalonians 2:13 (NKJV)**

Everybody loves a good transformation story.

I made it clear from the very beginning of sharing my story about finding freedom on my healthy living journey that you would not see pictures of bare midriffs on any of my online platforms.

Although I have helped women go from walking one mile to completing a 5K and others lose a significant amount of weight, their testimonials are always something like "I'm getting closer to God" or "I have more peace."

Why do they celebrate something like that, something you can't necessarily see in before and after pictures, instead of things like increased fitness level, weight loss, reduced cholesterol, and balanced blood sugars?

They have discovered that the secret to a sustainable healthy life is finding freedom in Christ.

Our lives, including our healthy lives, must be built on a foundation of faith.

My message is not merely faith and fitness. I do not simply share a scripture here and there while selling you a diet plan or program. I am here to share faith *then* fitness.

The approach is faith *first,* fitness *second*. I lead with God's Word. And God's Word transforms.

When we allow His truth about us to sink in, we live differently.

As a faith-filled woman, you want God to be first in your life. But you've likely been struggling so long in your body that it has consumed your thoughts and your energy. Ultimately, it's put you at odds with the One who created you.

I'm saying this because I lived it and I understand what's happening.

When you are at odds with your body and how you feel in it, you're at odds with your Creator. You have a hard time believing His Word about you, believing things like "You are fearfully and wonderfully made."

But God's Word transforms.

Whatever changes you are attempting to make in your life -- a habit you want to break or a goal you want to achieve -- seek God first.

Allow His Word to motivate you toward that which He is calling you. It may very well be a change that needs to take place physically, but until you allow His Word to penetrate your spirit, the physical changes will not mean as much.

## Action Step

This is your first step. You are beginning a journey that will lead you to a transformed life — mind, body, and spirit. Spend time in God's Word this week. Find a scripture that speaks to your situation. Make it your theme. Start working from the inside out.

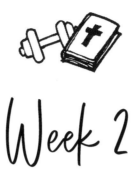

# Week 2

*Set your mind on things above, not on things on the earth.*

**Colossians 3:2 (NKJV)**

Where is your focus?

It is so easy to get caught up in the here and now. There's a to-do list that's as long as your arm. We live in a society that provides instant gratification. Social media easily draws us into the comparison trap.

It is too easy to get distracted. "Distracted driving" is a common phrase. And that's just driving. What about living?

When we are home with our families, we're distracted by the phone, the TV, the never-ending chore list. But this verse tells us something different.

*"Set your mind on things above."*

Things that matter. Things that last.

Yes, we are here on earth and there are things to do. If I don't do the laundry, my guys won't have clothes for work and school. We have to do our chores and pay attention to the to-do list BUT...

What drives and motivates must come from above.

Why are you doing what you're doing?

How do you know where you're focusing?

If it's not in the right place, how can you get back on track?

Where are you looking for praise and validation?

If your answers to these questions are something that can be gone tomorrow, then perhaps your focus needs to shift.

Take a break and spend time in God's Word.

### Action Step

Make daily quiet time a priority this week.

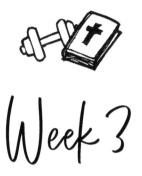

# Week 3

*Unless the Lord builds the house, they labor in vain who build it; Unless the Lord guards the city, the watchman keeps awake in vain.*

**Psalm 127:1 (NASB)**

Upon what are you building? Who is your builder?

Our focus needs to stay on Jesus.

Whether you are building a family, a business, a healthy life, a future, whatever you are doing, the key to it lasting and being worth anything is to build it on a firm foundation.

What is that foundation? Who is the One who knows how to lay that foundation?

It is Jesus.

You are ~~reading this devotional~~ here because you see the need to integrate your faith and your fitness.

A healthy life must be built on a foundation of faith.

We are not filling our bodies with healthy food in order to achieve a certain number on a scale. We are not drinking more water to detox. We are not moving more so that we can squeeze into a smaller pant size.

We are doing these things to honor the One who entrusted us with our bodies. We want to be the best version of ourselves *so* we can go out and be and do all that God has created us for.

We are building a fit life on a firm foundation. We are inviting Jesus to be part of this healthy living journey.

It is not the typical message you hear when you go searching for fitspiration. But we are not here to be *typical*.

We are here to be obedient to Jesus by grasping onto the power that is available to us to live the life He has called us to live.

Are you building on a firm foundation? Ask God to start laying the foundation.

## Action Step

Do a social media detox. Get rid of distractions and anything that will not enforce your firm foundation.

Week 3

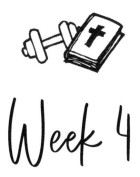

# Week 4

*Am I now trying to win the approval of human beings, or of God? Or am I trying to please people? If I were still trying to please people, I would not be a servant of Christ.*

**Galatians 1:10 (NIV)**

My early days of dieting and weight loss pursuit were all about gaining the approval of others. I did not want my mom to worry about my weight. In high school, I wanted the boys to notice me. When I got older, I wanted to gain the attention of someone to marry me.

Throughout that time, I compared myself to others and wanted to be as thin as so-and-so or look as good as so-and-so.

Eventually I had to admit that my obsession with weight loss was all about looking good to everyone around me. (Side note with a little tough love: People really didn't care how much I weighed, and they don't particularly care how much you do either. If they do, that is on them.)

I loved Jesus, but in this area of my life, I was not serving Him. I was serving myself. I was trying to please people and live up to what I thought society deemed thin and pretty and marriage worthy.

Thankfully, God did not give up on me.

When I grew tired of the constant pursuit of weight loss and excessive worry about what everyone thought, He was there to lead me in a new direction. I learned how to honor Him by honoring my body. That did not require a diet or a certain number on a scale. It simply required me to commit my healthy living journey to Him and let Him guide me.

Today is a good time to ask yourself why you do what you do. If no one is watching, are you still doing that thing, whatever that thing is?

If there is no one around to comment on your weight loss or your looks, will you still eat, move, exercise the way you were before no one was watching?

Is pleasing the Lord truly the motivation for your healthy living pursuit, whatever that looks like?

## Action Step

Write out your why. Keep asking why until you really drill it down to something very specific. For example, I want to get healthy. Why do you want to get healthy? I want to play with my grandchildren. Why do you want to play with your grandchildren? I want my grandchildren to have special memories of me throughout their lives.

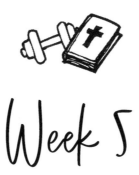

# Week 5

*Let us therefore come boldly to the throne of grace, that we may obtain mercy and find grace to help in time of need.*

**Hebrews 4:16 (NKJV)**

How do you approach the Lord? What concerns do you take to Him?

We can become timid with the Lord. We do not necessarily believe that everything — every single thing — is important to Him.

I have found myself using prayer as an afterthought. At times I will quickly make a decision and then later realize I should have prayed for direction before committing to or passing on something.

Some things seem too simple; maybe they wouldn't be important to the Lord. I run into this often when it comes to helping women with their fitness and body acceptance.

*Faith and fitness? How do those two things go together? You really pray about those things?*

They *do* go together. And yes, I pray about my relationship with my body as well as my relationships with food and exercise.

Most people consult the owner's manual of a new product to operate or assemble it. We have a Creator, a Maker. He wrote a book about how to live and filled it with the message of love for us.

Shouldn't we consult Him and that manual about everything? Even how to live in this body He has entrusted to us?

He invites us to come — and to come boldly — to His throne. You can approach Him and ask for His help in any and every situation.

In fact, that's the way He wants it. That's what He desires from us, to come to Him and lay our concerns at His feet. He will give us help.

What is your struggle this week? Is there something on your mind that you think you shouldn't bother Him with?

He is inviting you to come to His throne.

## Action Step

Go boldly to the Lord today and each day this week, Friend.

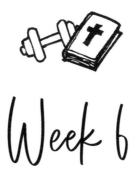

# Week 6

*He brought me to the banqueting house, and his banner over me was love.*

**Song of Solomon 2:4 (NKJV)**

The Song of Solomon is truly a love story, and it is in the Bible for two reasons. One reason is to teach us a few things to apply to our marriages. But the second and more important reason is to give us a glimpse of how the church is the bride of Christ and how much He loves us.

Before we can talk about love and how we are called to love others, you and I must accept Christ's love for us.

I have found in my own life that this is more difficult than it seems. I grew up singing "Jesus loves me this I know," but there was some disconnect. Yes, I knew that He loved me, but I did not fully accept His unconditional love.

I received Him into my heart and my life as a young girl, but years of body image struggles and insecurities kept me from fully embracing that love. Or rather, because I did not embrace that love, I lived many years with body image struggles and insecurities that I didn't need to.

Wasted time. Or so I thought.

Thankfully, no experience we have is wasted in the hands of God.

His banner over me is love. The bride does not have to fear or be nervous or self-conscious because she knows that her beloved loves her. She is confident in his love for her. She feels safe and protected by his love.

And so we can rest in Christ's love for us. His protective and undying and unconditional love for me and you - just as we are.

Look up. His banner over you is love.

## Action Step

Listen to the song "Jesus Loves Me." I guarantee it will stick in your mind all week.

Week 6

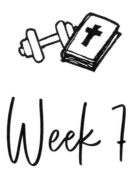

# Week 7

*Thus says the Lord: "Stand in the ways and see, and ask for the old paths, where the good way is, and walk in it; Then you will find rest for your souls. But they said, 'We will not walk in it.'"*

### Jeremiah 6:16 (NKJV)

It is not often that we are told to look back or to go the old way, but when we get off course or become distracted, that is exactly what we must do.

In this passage, Jeremiah is telling the Israelites that they need to return to their faith, the faith that they learned from Moses and those before them, and to follow it.

Unfortunately, they chose not to.

Let us apply this to our healthy living journey. Where are you on that path? Are you looking for motivation to move? Have you been searching for a diet plan to help you lose weight? Do you find yourself unsettled in this area of your life and constantly trying something new?

What if I told you that you will have to go back to your beginning to find the answer?

*You were fearfully and wonderfully made.* (See Psalm 139.) When you were born, you listened to your body and let someone know when you were hungry, and you likely let them know when you were full. You moved your body freely and rested when needed.

Over time it became complicated. You lost touch with your natural instincts. You got distracted by things you saw around you. You likely began comparing and striving for more, for a different version of yourself.

And if you are like me, you may have taken God out of the equation. You might have started thinking He was not interested in you anymore. You may have felt like He somehow got it wrong when He created you like this.

Those are lies the enemy would want us to believe. It is how he distracts us from fully receiving God's love for us and living the life He's called us to live.

Today He is telling you that the good way is to get back on the path where you believed what He said about you. He wants you to return to those times when you simply honored the unique body He entrusted to you.

It is the only place you will find rest from this struggle.

## Action Step

Look back to the beginning when God created you. Find a baby picture and reflect on your life. God created you with a plan and a purpose.

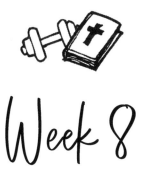

# Week 8

*As you therefore have received Christ Jesus the Lord, so walk in Him, rooted and built up in Him and established in the faith, as you have been taught, abounding in it with thanksgiving.*

**Colossians 2:6-7 (NKJV)**

Rooted in Christ.

Everything originates from the roots. The trees spring forth out of the ground but not before their roots have gone down deep. They go deep to get water and minerals to grow.

It is in Christ and through Him that we become strong and can walk into the life He has for us.

Why faith and fitness?

I think this verse is a good place to start. If we are in Christ, we must walk in Him and build our entire lives on Him. Our lives are established in faith in Christ.

To me, that means everything I do, all that I am, the big and the small things must be built on that firm foundation. It all needs to be rooted in Christ.

For too long, I built parts of my life on Christ, but other parts, like my body image struggles, I just could not let those go.

But then I finally let Him take that part of me too. I realized that all of it, everything in my life must be built firmly on Him and established in the faith.

Are there any areas you are holding back? Any areas where you are struggling?

Is it time to give it all to Him and then be grateful for what He is going to do and the new growth that will come?

## Action Step

Plant something this week. Let it be a reminder that something must take root to grow.

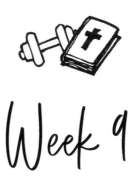

# Week 9

*"For I will restore health to you and heal you of your wounds," says the Lord.*

**Jeremiah 30:17a (NKJV)**

Whether your motivation for a healthier lifestyle is to get in better shape or to help you battle a life-threatening illness, God wants to heal you.

Many people commit to getting healthy at the beginning of the year. Most New Year's resolutions include things like lose weight, eat better, start an exercise program.

Those are all great intentions, but when they stand alone, outside of the overall picture of your life, they are bound to fail.

God is our Creator and therefore He is our Helper and our Healer. He is the one who knows how we need to live our lives, including eating and exercising. He knows what is best for our bodies.

Oftentimes our goals of becoming healthier are the result of a lack of self-care. Over time people tend to fall into habits that are not so good for them.

God wants to restore us. He wants to get us back to a healthy version of ourselves so that we can live the life He has called us to live.

It is difficult to accomplish His business when we lack energy and stamina and when we do not feel good about ourselves.

I don't know where you are on your healthy living journey. But if you feel like you have fallen off the wagon or gotten off track, God wants to restore you to health.

If you are fighting a battle of deteriorating health due to a severe illness or disease, God is your Healer. I don't know how He will choose to heal you, but I know He can, and He will in His way and in His time.

No matter where you are this week and what kind of healing or restoration you need, know that your Creator knows exactly what you need and is ready to heal and restore you.

We serve a mighty God!

## Action Step

Spend time with your Healer each day this week. Implement one new healthy habit and practice it daily.

# Week 10

*Let this mind be in you which was also in Christ Jesus...*

**Philippians 2:5 (NKJV)**

We cannot escape our thoughts.

I don't know about you, but my mind can be an unwelcome place. Thoughts and ideas tend to pop in unannounced and then stay there. Other times I get focused on a negative event or negative words and cannot let it go.

Destructive thoughts can take over quickly. I know that is not the mind of Christ. But how can I have the mind of Christ?

If you have found yourself with the same battle in your mind, know that you are not alone. There is hope. There is a way to "let this mind be in you which was also in Christ Jesus."

It starts by filling your mind with His Word. Daily Bible reading, scripture memorization, and prayer are all actions that will make your mind a more welcoming place to be.

The Bible is filled with God's thoughts on you as well as His thoughts on how to live your life.

It is easy to get distracted by setting our minds on the here and now. Our thoughts focus on what's right in front of us or what has us troubled. Those things gain our full attention. Doing so only keeps us in a cycle of defeat and constant battle in our minds.

A war is waging in your mind, but let Christ in and you can win that war.

Does your mind focus on negative thoughts and feelings toward your body? Do you worry about weight and plan everything around how to lose that weight?

If you are struggling to implement healthy habits that you can stick with, head to God's Word. He has so much to say to you.

Until you start looking at yourself through the lens of His Word, you will not stick with a plan that is sustainable.

Anything you want to change in your life on the outside will only change when you start by addressing what is going on inside in your mind.

"Let this mind be in you which was also in Christ Jesus," then your circumstance will begin to change too.

## Action Step

Fill your mind with Christ. Pick a scripture to memorize this week.

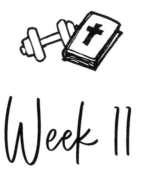

# Week 11

*As the Scriptures say, "People are like grass; their beauty is like a flower in the field. The grass withers and the flower fades. But the word of the Lord remains forever." And that word is the Good News that was preached to you.*

**1 Peter 1:24-25 (NLT)**

How is it that we have bought into the lies that our life's purpose is to lose weight, that we must pursue beauty at all costs?

And what is beauty anyway? By society's standards, it is a young, thin body.

But here's the deal: We all age, and with age comes change, whether you're a person or a flower. In fact, the alternative of aging is, well, not being here at all.

Other translations of the verse above use words like "droops and dries up." That made me chuckle as I thought of this scripture in relation to our aging bodies. If you are beyond your mid-40s like I am, I imagine you're familiar with words like drooping, fading, and withering when it comes to your body!

But this is a serious matter. What are you pursuing? Are you pursuing the world's standards of beauty more than you are pursuing Christ?

Everyone ages. As part of that process, we change. It is the way God made it to be. For flowers. For grass. And for people.

You and I will eventually fade away. It is called the cycle of life.

So do we spend our days in constant pursuit of weight loss only to feel frustrated at every corner?

Or do we pursue the Lord and simply be a good steward of what He has entrusted us with?

I believe He wants us to pursue Him. In doing so, we will also pursue health and wellness but not at the cost of our focus on Him. Instead, it will be in a way that honors Him.

So while the messages around us trend toward beauty at all costs, let us choose to listen to God's Word and allow His message to guide us to what He wants us to pursue.

## Action Step

Buy a bouquet of flowers this week. Let them serve as a reminder of this verse.

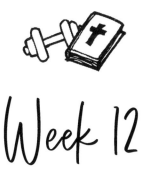

# Week 12

*If any of you lacks wisdom, let him ask of God, who gives to all liberally and without reproach, and it will be given to him.*

**James 1:5 (NKJV)**

Is it that we think we have got this? Or do we not even think to ask?

I don't know about you, but I cannot remember the last time I asked for wisdom. Is it because I think I have it all together and do not need any? Not a chance.

All too often, asking for wisdom in a situation, big or small, is (I hate to admit it) one of the last things I do instead of the first.

But if I am not asking for wisdom, then maybe my ugly pride is making me think I am okay and I have got this after all.

That is no fun to admit, but here in God's Word we are told if you lack wisdom, just ask for it!

My healthy living journey is a great example of how I should have asked for wisdom a lot sooner than I did.

I prayed and prayed that God would help me with the body image battle and weight loss struggle, but I did not truly ask for (and listen to!) the wisdom He could provide me.

God knows our bodies better than we do. He created us! When it comes to figuring out how to live a healthy life that is sustainable, we need His wisdom.

He can help you learn to listen to your body and the cues it gives you about how to take care of it. Each one of us is different, and we need to honor that.

I do not know what your struggle is. It may be healthy living or it may be a job concern or a relationship issue. But I do know that God wants to guide you through it.

Will you take a moment and admit that you do not have all the answers and ask Him to give you wisdom today?

## Action Step

Ask God's guidance and seek out guidance from someone who is farther along on their faith and fitness journey.

Week 12

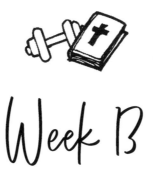

# Week 13

*And let us consider how we may spur one another on toward love and good deeds, not giving up meeting together, as some are in the habit of doing, but encouraging one another — and all the more as you see the Day approaching.*

**Hebrews 10:24-25 (NIV)**

We need each other.

The Bible is clear about our need for community. God recognized it at Creation when He said it was not good for man to be alone. (See Genesis 2:18.)

I considered myself a loner when I was growing up. In fact, it was a label people put on me at an early age, so I thought that was how I was supposed to be.

My plan was to go through life mostly on my own, keeping to

myself, and not getting close to many people.

But going through life alone is hard. It is not healthy to hold onto your struggles by yourself. Burdens are heavier and accomplishments are not as meaningful when you are celebrating alone.

We are not fine all the time. And that is okay. We are not supposed to be. But we do need people in our lives to encourage us, to support us, to pray for us, and to spur us along.

We are called to be there for one another. The only way we can help each other is to get together and commit to traveling this journey alongside one another.

No matter where you are on your journey, please do not go another step alone. Find your tribe. Connect with someone. I know it is tough. I know it can be scary to reach out and to become vulnerable, but God will bless you for it.

It has made such a difference in my life. I became more confident. I let go of some of my weight loss worries. I got healthier in my mind and my body.

You can do that too.

## Action Step

Find your tribe. Connect with someone. If you need suggestions, go to the Epilogue on page 213 to learn how you can connect with me.

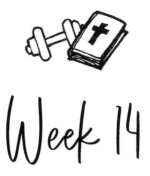

# Week 14

*It is for freedom that Christ has set us free. Stand firm, then, and do not let yourselves be burdened again by a yoke of slavery.*

**Galatians 5:1 (NIV)**

Diets. Quick fixes. Negative body image. Worries about weight and the reflection in the mirror.

These things consumed my mind and my thoughts starting as early as fifth grade and well into my adult life. I used my time and money to try anything that promised weight loss, especially a flat belly!

Every morning I prayed about this struggle. I read God's Word and wrote verses on note cards, but then I spent the rest of my day feeling insecure, worrying about how I looked, wondering what the number would be on the scale that day, and searching for a new diet that promised to help me lose the pounds once and for all.

I was a slave to the pursuit of weight loss. I was bound up by worry and anxiety, all because of how I viewed my body. I wanted to be free. I desperately wanted to find freedom from this struggle.

I knew God could set me free. He wanted to set me free. It is why He came to earth, to set you and me free from whatever it is that holds us back from His best for our lives.

However, I would not let go — until I did.

I found that freedom, or rather finally accepted that freedom, about nine years ago.

But here is the thing. It is something I must pursue daily. If you have ever felt that bondage, I imagine you know what I mean.

This struggle, these worries, they still show up.

Do you see the middle of this verse? "Do not let yourselves be burdened again…"

When the old ways of thinking come or when I find myself clicking on a weight loss link or feeling insecure because of something I see on social media, I feel the Holy Spirit say, "Not again. You have been set free. You don't want to carry that burden again."

So I remind myself of where I was and how God has set me free. And then I take a step in the direction of freedom, not backward to bondage.

What is it for you? Do you need to be set free? God can do it.

Have you been set free but have recently felt the pull back into the struggle? Choose today to stand firm in His freedom.

> ## Action Step
> Get honest with yourself. Have you gone back to some old ways of thinking or doing things? Ask God to set you free.

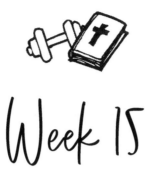

# Week 15

*And Jesus cried out again with a loud voice, and yielded up His spirit. Then, behold, the veil of the temple was torn in two from top to bottom; and the earth quaked, and the rocks were split...*

### Matthew 27:50-51 (NKJV)

Matthew 27:50 records Jesus' last breath. He cried out and then yielded up His Spirit.

Let us pause for a moment and consider that. He yielded up His Spirit. He willingly surrendered for you and me. He died.

And the result of that brings us to verse 51. It is one of my favorite moments in scripture. Jesus dies, and at that very minute, the veil in the temple was torn.

This veil was not like a curtain sheer. It was a very heavy curtain that, according to scripture, separated the Most Holy Place, the place where God's presence was found, from the rest of the temple.

This is our visual of what Christ's death did for us.

Because of His death and resurrection we have direct access to our Heavenly Father. We can call on Him, and He hears us.

There is no need for sacrifice and burnt offerings. All He asks is that we humbly come to Him. The door to Him is open. His arms are open to receive you.

Oh what a privilege we have to be in the Father's presence! We have access to a Savior who loves us more than we can comprehend. There is nothing left to separate us from His love.

Run into His arms today.

## Action Step

Place some Easter decorations in a place where you will see them every day and remind yourself of what Jesus did for you on the cross.

Week 15

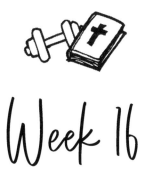

# Week 16

*Now the Lord is the Spirit; and where the Spirit of the Lord is, there is liberty.*

## 2 Corinthians 3:17 (NKJV)

Several months ago, I was struggling. I felt like I was going backward, back to the days when weight loss worries plagued my mind, back to the days when I questioned everything about myself - my looks, my body, my running, how I was doing as a wife and mother.

I simply felt "off."

But then the Holy Spirit led me to this verse. Where the Spirit of the Lord is, there is freedom.

I was feeling everything but freedom. In fact, I felt like I was back to my days of wandering that desert and feeling bound by weight loss worries and insecurities in every area of my life.

So I had to ask myself, "Is Christ first in my life? Am I fully surrendered?"

I had allowed things to get out of order in my life.

Thankfully the Lord is always available to us. He is ready to assume first place in our lives once we allow Him to. You see, He never pushes Himself on us. We must *choose* to give Him the top spot.

I don't like me or my life when He's not first and when I'm not surrendered to Him. When I start to feel something other than freedom, I ask myself, "Am I allowing the Spirit of the Lord to rule in my life?"

You can be sure that I take a moment to lay it at His feet yet again. I do not want to operate any other way. How about you? Are you experiencing freedom in your life? If not, that can change with a simple prayer.

## Action Step

Are you experiencing freedom in your life? Meditate on this question this week during your quiet time and talk to God about any feelings that are not associated with His freedom.

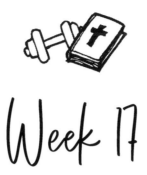

# Week 17

*Why spend your money on food that does not give you strength? Why pay for food that does you no good? Listen to me, and you will eat what is good. You will enjoy the finest food.*

**Isaiah 55:2 (NLT)**

I hate to think about all of the money I spent on trying to lose weight.

I bought every diet pill, plan, book, program, magazine, shake, supplement that offered even the slightest promise of weight loss. Add to it even the smallest hope of losing belly fat, and I was all in, skip the 30-day supply and go straight for 90 days!

Hot-Pants, anyone?

"Just wear these spandex-like shorts to bed and your waist will magically shrink overnight." I fell for it.

I was searching for and spending money on false promises. I

made healthy living much more difficult *and way more expensive* than it was intended to be.

The pursuit was part of a larger problem that I had to eventually admit: I needed more of Jesus in my life.

I needed to pursue Him. I needed to believe what He said about me in His Word. I needed to feed on His Word to heal my relationship with my body. And the great thing about consuming His Word is it does not cost any money. It is free.

His gift of new life is free to us. He paid all our debts. We can consume the fine food of His Word and the wonderful truths about who we are and *whose* we are.

Ask God to give you a hunger that only He can satisfy. When you eat from His table, you will gain a better perspective of how to care for your physical body.

Stop the Google searches, step away from the computer, put away your credit card, and invest some time in God's Word this week.

### Action Step

Take a day off from social media this week. Spend your time browsing God's Word. Commit to a spending break.

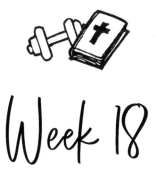

# Week 18

*Two are better than one, because they have a good reward for their labor. For if they fall, one will lift up his companion. But woe to him who is alone when he falls, for he has no one to help him up.*

### Ecclesiastes 4:9-10 (NKJV)

I know what it is like to be surrounded by people and still feel alone.

There have been several different times in my life when I felt very alone, even when I was surrounded with friends and family. One of those times was a very long period when I struggled with my reflection in the mirror.

I did not feel like anyone understood what I was going through, and more importantly, I didn't want to admit that I was struggling with this.

On the outside things seemed fine. In school, I was near the top of my class. In my marriage, I showed up with a smile on my face.

But I was still fighting the battles in my mind - alone. Yes, I prayed to God and I read His Word, but I still felt so alone.

Thankfully, I have learned along the way that I wasn't meant to journey alone. We were not meant to do this life, any of it, on our own.

To be sure, we need God as our source of strength and support. But He has also made us need each other.

This verse in Ecclesiastes serves as a reminder that two are better than one and if (or when!) we fall, that friend is there to lift us up. Do you have real relationships and experience community with your friends and family, or do you find yourself in a room full of people feeling lonely?

Friend, you do not have to be alone. You were not meant to.

Reach out to a friend. Plan to take a walk or enjoy a cup of coffee together. Take time to connect with others.

*Action Step*

...Now what I am commanding you today is not too difficult...

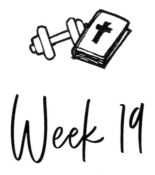

# Week 19

*for you or beyond your reach.*

**Deuteronomy 30:11 (NIV)**

L ife is hard.

But is it?

Yes, we have trials and tribulations. Everyone has struggles and difficulties, sometimes unimaginable roads to travel. But there are times when we humans make things difficult that do not need to be made so difficult.

Life is not too hard.

In this week's scripture, God was speaking through Moses to

His people about the commandments He was giving them.

We do not serve a God who is sitting in Heaven trying to trip us up. He is not calculating all the ways that He can make us fail. He wants the best for you and me. The things He asks of us are things He equips us for.

The commandments that He gives are within our reach. We can do this! I have been on this healthy living journey my entire life, and I've been helping women along the way for several years. One thing I have learned: We make it hard. We complicate it when it does not need to be that way.

Caring for our bodies should not be difficult. It becomes difficult when we attempt to consume all the information and try every diet, gimmick, and quick fix that is out there.

But God has given us the Holy Spirit and an intelligent mind that simply needs to get in tune with our own body by first embracing who He has created us to be.

A healthy life. Freedom in mind and body. Acceptance of yourself. Peace. It is all within reach when you approach it the way God intends.

If the way that you are pursuing health seems too hard, then it is time to reconsider your methods. If you are not experiencing peace and freedom, then perhaps it is time to invite the Holy Spirit to guide you.

Start with God's Word and learn the truth about yourself.

We have enough difficult things to deal with. Do not make obedience to God in your everyday, healthy life be one of those things. He did not intend it to be too difficult.

## Action Step

Discard the list of food rules you have been conditioned to follow and identify three simple things you can do each day to support your healthy life. For example, drink more water, eat protein at every meal, and take a short walk.

A Year of Sundays

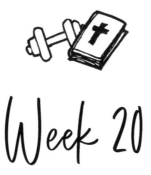

# Week 20

*She gave this name to the Lord who spoke to her: "You are the God who sees me," for she said, "I have now seen the One who sees me."*

**Genesis 16:13 (NIV)**

Hagar was rejected. She felt alone. But God never left her. He was there.

He is always there. God saw Hagar, and He sees you.

It sounds so simple, and on the one hand, it is.

God sees us.

He sees you.

He sees me.

That is just the way He is.

He is a loving God who is concerned about His creation, you and me.

While simple, this truth is also profound. It is huge. It is amazing and nearly unfathomable that God in Heaven *does* see you and me.

I don't know about you, but I find it difficult to wrap my mind around this some days, to grasp that the God of the universe sees insignificant little ol' me.

Have you felt that way too?

It's easy to dismiss ourselves and feel unworthy or not enough. But I want you to know that there is nothing insignificant about you.

You are worthy.

You are known.

You are enough.

You are loved.

He sees you.

## Action Step

Take a moment and sit quietly. Envision your Heavenly Father looking down on you right now, not with judgment but with adoring eyes, eyes only for you. Let the moment wash over you and envelop you with the comfort and safety of His love.

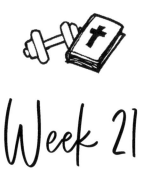

# Week 21

*We are hard-pressed on every side, yet not crushed; we are perplexed, but not in despair; persecuted, but not forsaken; struck down, but not destroyed — always carrying about in the body the dying of the Lord Jesus, that the life of Jesus also may be manifested in our body.*

### 2 Corinthians 4:8-10 (NKJV)

It seems like the devil likes to attack women through weight loss worries and ongoing struggles with body image. I imagine that struggle was something that drew you to this book.

Early in my life, the enemy found that those were the easy targets to get me down and distracted and keep me that way.

You see, all the devil wants to do is get us to take our eyes off Jesus and get them on ourselves. And Satan does a good job of attacking and distracting.

Even when I thought I was trying to change my outlook and

do things "right," I would struggle and fall again.

The enemy has a plan to get us down. He will take whatever weakness we have and magnify it to distract us from God's voice in our lives.

I fell under that pressure many times, but because of Christ in me, I did not stay down. I could not stay down. His Holy Spirit in me would not allow me to be overtaken by Satan's tactics. I had to seek God's help and call on His name. He heard me. He helped me.

God still helps me fight this battle because the devil does not stop trying to get us down. He will use whatever he can.

But you and I, we have Jesus Christ in us. We have victory because He already defeated Satan and all his schemes.

No matter what your struggle is, it is not going to destroy you. Jesus is on your side. His life is in you to help you.

In fact, this verse gives us the confidence that the life of Jesus is to be manifested in our bodies. He lives in us and works through us.

Instead of allowing weight loss worries and body image struggles distract us, let us allow them to bring us closer to Jesus. Seek His Word and the truth He says about you, then remind the devil who you are and whose you are.

Will you reach up and take hold of Christ's hand today and let Him lift you up so you can stand for Him?

## Action Step

Speak an affirmation out loud, such as "I am loved." Repeat it daily this week.

# Week 22

*Therefore, as God's chosen people, holy and dearly loved, clothe yourselves with compassion, kindness, humility, gentleness and patience. Bear with each other and forgive one another if any of you has a grievance against someone. Forgive as the Lord forgave you. And over all these virtues put on love, which binds them all together in perfect unity. Let the peace of Christ rule in your hearts, since as members of one body you were called to peace. And be thankful.*

**Colossians 3:12-15 (NIV)**

What are you wearing?

Most of the time, you will find me in comfortable casual clothes — shorts, T-shirts, sweatshirts, yoga pants. If I'm "dressing up," it's jeans!

What I am comfortable in and what makes me feel good may

be very different from your style, and that's okay.

I am no fashionista, and that's why this week's devotion has nothing to do with what you're wearing on your body. This is about what God wants us to wear. He has a dress code for us.

Wear compassion, kindness, humility, gentleness, patience, forgiveness. He even tells us what type of "overcoat" to wear: Love.

When we dress like this, peace begins to rule in our hearts, and this leads to gratitude.

Now, more than ever, we need to be concerned about what we are clothing ourselves with daily. People are watching. God has placed us among friends, family, and strangers. They need us to be compassionate and kind and patient. We cannot be those things on our own.

Daily we need to go to God's closet — His Word — to dress appropriately.

The overcoat of love.

The world needs His love. You can be the one to share that with others when you dress the way He desires for you to.

You may not be going to a worship service today, but you can still take some time to dress for the Savior.

## Action Step

As you get dressed every day this week, think of this verse. Ask yourself which qualities you want to wear that day.

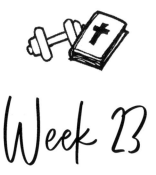

# Week 23

*And let the beauty of the Lord our God be upon us, and establish the work of our hands for us; Yes, establish the work of our hands.*

**Psalm 90:17 (NKJV)**

From an early age, the pursuit of beauty seems to be top of mind for every female. Over the years, we do all the things that we believe will make us beautiful. The retail market even refers to make-up and other skin care products as "beauty products."

And what about all the diets a woman will try over her lifetime in the name of improving her look?

Yet all the while, we simply need to surrender to the Lord.

Let the beauty of the Lord our God be upon us.

When I read words like "let" and "upon us," I envision a

covering. I picture pausing and allowing the Lord to blanket me with His beauty.

We need only allow Him to put His beauty on us.

He created you. You are the way you are supposed to be. There is no need to pursue all the things in order to be called beautiful by another's standards.

What God desires is that you pursue Him and the life He has designed for you to live. He does not want you to become distracted by the pursuit of fleeting beauty.

When we surrender to Him, He will cover us with His beauty.

Isn't the most beautiful person that you encounter the one who is living confidently, doing the thing God has called her to do?

Aren't you most beautiful when you can look at yourself in the mirror with confidence, certain that you are living the life Christ designed for you?

Beauty begins on the inside with a heart surrendered to the Lord. Then, and only then, is it reflected on the outside. And that beauty has nothing to do with the smoothness of your skin, the number on the scale, or the clothes that you wear.

Let the beauty of the Lord our God be upon you this week.

## Action Step

When you stand in front of the mirror this week, look for the beauty of the Lord.

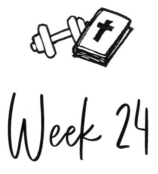

# Week 24

*But blessed is the one who trusts in the Lord, whose confidence is in him.*

**Jeremiah 17:7 (NIV)**

Confidence comes when we know not only *who* we are but also *whose* we are.

Dictionary.com defines confidence as *"belief in oneself."* But we are nothing without Christ. Therefore, we only gain true and lasting confidence when we first trust in the Lord.

When we find ourselves suffering from a lack of confidence, we must ask ourselves where our trust is.

Are you relying on your looks or your level of success to make you feel confident?

Do you think losing a few pounds or gaining a new position at work will improve your confidence?

Are you looking to a person or a relationship to give you confidence?

Our relationship with the Lord is the only steady and reliable thing that we have. Our confidence starts there.

Because of Him, we can have assurance that we are enough. Because His Word says it, we can believe that we were created in His image.

That makes you and me special.

When you believe that you are enough and that you are special, your confidence grows.

Anything you build must be set on a firm foundation. And the only firm foundation I know is the Lord.

Confidence comes from putting our trust in the Lord. That is the first step. *Then* commit to daily trusting Him and believing what He says about you.

If you want more confidence, ask yourself where you are placing your trust. Placing it in anything but the Lord will leave you lacking and unsure.

Turn to His Word today and start building your firm foundation.

Use positive statements:

*I am enough.*

*God loves me just the way I am.*

*I am valuable.*

*I have been created in the image of God.*

Do you want to build confidence? Put your trust in Jesus.

## Action Step

Surround yourself with positive words. Consider purchasing a bracelet with those words on it. Check out Momentum Jewelry (https://momentumjewelry.com) for ideas.

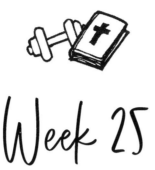

# Week 25

*Therefore I tell you, do not worry about your life, what you will eat or drink; or about your body, what you will wear. Is not life more than food, and the body more than clothes? Look at the birds of the air; they do not sow or reap or store away in barns, and yet your heavenly Father feeds them. Are you not much more valuable than they?*

Matthew 6:25-26 (NIV)

"Is not life more than food, and the body more than clothes?"

Mic drop!

There are days I need someone to ask me this question then make me sit with it.

There was a time in my life, a very long time, that the only thing my life hinged on was what I would eat, how I looked in my clothes, and what I needed to do to lose weight so I could wear a smaller size.

I ignored the care and concern the Father took to create me in a unique way that was beautiful to Him. I dismissed His unconditional love for me. I overlooked the blessings in my life because the only thing I could focus on was what I saw wrong with myself.

We need to be good stewards of our bodies because we need to be healthy to fulfill the calling God has placed on our lives, but that does not require us to present a certain outward image. It only requires a heart surrendered to Him, a heart that trusts Him with all we are.

Are you spending more time reading food labels than reading the Bible?

Do you spend more time studying and researching the latest diet trends than studying scripture?

Are you more focused on the size of your jeans than on the person in front of you who needs you to show them Christ's love?

People do not care what you're wearing or what you ate for breakfast. Instead, people need to see Jesus in you. Isn't that what we are called to do? Be Jesus to others. Show them He loves them exactly like they are, as He does you.

The last piece of the verse: *"Are you not much more valuable than they (the birds of the air)?"*

God values you. He loves you.

Live loved this week.

> ## Action Step
> 
> Get outside every day this week. Go for a nature walk. Notice God's beauty around you.

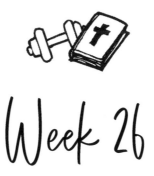

# Week 26

*You were getting along so well. Who has interfered with you to hold you back from following the truth? It certainly isn't God who has done it, for he is the one who has called you to freedom in Christ. But it takes only one wrong person among you to infect all the others.*

### Galatians 5:7-9 (TLB)

When I read this verse, I wanted to jump up and down and shout, "This! This right here!"

In fact, when I was writing this devotional entry, my fingers were flying across my keyboard. I want you to feel the passion behind this message and the words in this verse.

Let's look at the New Living Translation of this passage:

"You were running the race so well. Who has held you back from following the truth? It certainly is not God, for he is the one who called you to freedom. This false teaching is like a little yeast that spreads through the whole batch of dough!"

It is time to get honest about your relationship with food and your body.

Whether you are like me and started this cycle of struggle with your weight and body image at a young age or it happened later in life for you, there was a time you were going along (running your race) feeling good in your body. You had a good relationship with food. All until this was not the case.

At what point did someone or something plant a seed that you were not good enough? When did you stop believing that you are fearfully and wonderfully made? What made you think that you must look a certain way to be loved?

When did you get distracted by the noise that said you must be on a diet and pursue weight loss to be accepted?

Where did this thinking come from? It has been planted in our minds from society and likely from real people in our lives who have judged us.

Those behind the multimillion-dollar diet business, many who try to disguise themselves as advocates for health and wellness, are the false teachers who spread misinformation to men and women of all ages. And nothing makes my heart break more.

Friend, you were running the race so well. What happened?

Please hear this: You do not have to lose weight to prove your worth. You can stop comparing yourself to others and be you.

God has something special for you right now, and He does not require you to look a certain way to live the life He has designed for you.

You can break free from dieting and feel good in your body. You can be fit and healthy *and* be free.

And here is the best part: You can get back into the race and run it well. You do not have to stay stuck in a place of defeat. You can shift your focus from diets and learn the truth of who God says you are and how He wants you to care for your unique body.

## Action Step

Do you feel like you have taken some steps backward? Are you at a plateau, not growing in your faith or pursuing healthy habits? Set aside some time this week to dig deep. Ask the hard questions. Take inventory. Ask God to search your heart. Identify where things got off track and commit to fixing your eyes on Jesus and honoring Him by honoring your body.

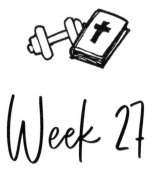

# Week 27

*It was good for me to be afflicted so that I might learn your decrees.*

### Psalm 119:71 (NIV)

Who likes to endure struggle, pain, and hardship?

I'm not raising my hand.

When you are right in the middle of affliction of any kind, it can be difficult to see good. And many times, it remains difficult to see the good even on the other side.

In today's verse, the psalmist declares that his struggle was good.

This verse makes me think of my own weight loss and body

image struggles. Without a doubt, this is what brought me to my knees — in the best of ways.

I know that might sound minor compared to all the pain and hardship people have experienced, but this affliction, if you will, started at a very young age and lasted many years.

I don't know how many tears I cried asking for this struggle and constant worry to go away. I didn't want to essentially fight with myself about how I looked.

My heart's desire was to feel good in my skin and to not worry about my weight. Once I finally allowed God to set me free, I was able to see the purpose in that struggle.

He did not make this affliction happen, but He allowed it.

Because of my struggle with weight and body image, not only did I learn how to live a healthy life in the way I eat and move, but I also have been given the opportunity to help other women find their own freedom from these struggles.

Instead of resenting an affliction you have experienced, how can you look at it and find good?

How is God using it in your life or in the lives of others?

Is it time for you to view your affliction in light of God's Word and how it can draw you and others closer to Him?

I pray that I am a good steward with my experiences, and I pray that you will be too. His ultimate goal is that you and I know Him more.

## Action Step

What is your struggle? Make a list of the positive things that have come from your struggle.

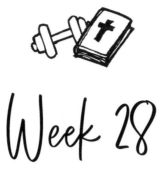

# Week 28

*I have set the Lord always before me; because He is at my right hand I shall not be moved.*

**Psalm 16:8 (NKJV)**

"Drishti" is a term used in yoga. Sometimes an instructor will say, "Find your drishti."

What is a drishti? Simply put, it is an immovable spot upon which to fix your gaze. The instructor often uses this cue when you are doing a pose that requires balance.

How do you find your drishti? Look ahead and find an immovable spot. Fix your gaze on that.

Why do you need a drishti? It helps you achieve better alignment and gives you a focus to concentrate on.

It is hard to find balance. Whether you are trying to find balance standing on one leg or trying to find balance in your crazy life, things can get wobbly. Sometimes you feel like there is no way you can remain standing.

Oftentimes, when I take my focus off my drishti in a yoga class, I immediately start swaying and fall out of the pose.

Do I even have to tell you what happens in life when you start looking at everything you must do while desperately trying to find balance?

Jesus is your drisht. He is where you need to set your focus. He is immovable.

When we keep our eyes on Jesus, we will stand firm. He will balance us. He will bring things into alignment in our lives. A focus on Jesus will give you intention.

Are your eyes fixed on something that moves? Are you looking at yourself or your circumstances?

Set your eyes on Jesus this week.

## Action Step

Practice your balance this week. Stand on one leg. Find an instructional video about the Tree Pose and try it.

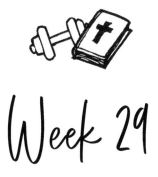

# Week 29

*Teach me to do Your will, for You are my God; Your Spirit is good. Lead me in the land of uprightness.*

**Psalm 143:10 (NKJV)**

If you are new to prayer or if you are new to morning quiet times, start with this passage. Read this scripture to the Lord. Make it your daily prayer.

If you have one of those days when you do not know where to go in your Bible or what to pray, use this.

Each day we have a new opportunity to learn what God wants us to do. He will give us a fresh glimpse of where He wants us to go.

How we start our day makes all the difference in the rest of it.

Each day may not go exactly as you planned, but it will go

exactly as the Lord intends as long as you give it to Him.

Are you giving Him your days? Are you starting with a teachable spirit and a heart surrendered to Him?

> ## Action Step
>
> Make Psalm 143:10 your prayer every day this week.

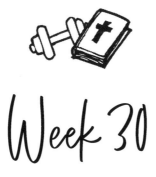

# Week 30

*But blessed is the one who trusts in the Lord, whose confidence is in him.*

**Jeremiah 17:7 (NIV)**

I am enough.

It is a familiar affirmation. I have a Momentum Jewelry bracelet with this saying on it. I even have a reminder set on my phone to remind me of this.

But on my own, I am not enough.

When I say I am enough, I say it only because of Christ in me.

With Christ, I am enough.

With Christ, you are enough.

*Because of* Christ in me, I am enough.

I have all I need *when* my hope and my trust are in Him.

On my own, no way. Cannot do it. Will not do it.

*I need Him.*

I confidently say "I am enough" because my trust is in the Lord.

What about you? Do you feel like you are enough?

If you are struggling with this, ask yourself where you are putting your hope and trust.

Without Him, we are nothing. We cannot do it.

But with Christ, we have all that we need.

You and I, Christ in us, we are enough.

### Action Step

Set a reminder on your phone or put a Post-it note on your computer that says "I am enough."

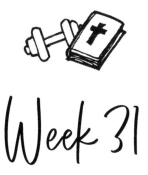

# Week 31

*Cast all your anxiety on him because he cares for you.*

**1 Peter 5:7 (NIV)**

Worry. Anxiety. Fear. Do you have any?

If you are like me, I know that you do.

Too often I carry anxiety, fear, and worry about big things, little things, and all the things in between. Many times it is because I feel I need to control situations and outcomes.

Sometimes I think that if I do not concern myself over it, no one else will. But the truth is, God does care. He cares about me and everything that is happening in my life - the little things and the big things and all the things in between.

He cares for you too. He cares about all those things in your life.

I found written in my Bible margin next to this verse: *You are God's only care and concern.*

Friend, He loves you. He wants nothing more than to carry that burden for you. He does not want to see you bogged down by the weight of worry, fear, and anxiety. We are carrying these things unnecessarily.

He is there waiting for you to toss it to Him. Let Him carry it.

It is time for you — and me — to let that thing go and not be hindered and held back.

Will you spend some time with the Lord today and give Him your concerns so you can walk in the freedom that He has already bought for you?

You are His only concern today. Let Him care for you.

### Action Step

Take your cares to the Lord daily this week. Nothing is too big or too insignificant for our God.

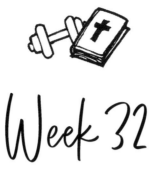

# Week 32

*Not what goes into the mouth defiles a man; but what comes out of the mouth, this defiles a man.*

### Matthew 15:11 (NKJV)

In this passage in Matthew 15, the scribes noticed that Jesus' disciples ate bread without washing their hands and determined that this defiled them.

Jesus corrected the scribes' thinking by telling them that it is not what goes into the mouth that defiles the man but what comes out.

I spent lots of years analyzing everything I ate, how many calories I ate, when I should eat, etc. My focus was on everything that went into my mouth in hopes that I would find the right formula to help me lose weight. All the while, I was not concerned with what was coming out of my mouth.

Because of my focus on what was going in, I was critical of myself and others. I was caught in comparison and competition. I was never happy because I was always focusing on food and how I could eat to lose weight.

My heart was not in a good place, and therefore the things coming out of my mouth were not always uplifting and encouraging.

Should we be concerned over what we put into our bodies? Yes. We need to be good stewards of the one body we have each been given.

However, the condition of our hearts is not measured by how fast or far we can run or what the number is on a scale. It is evident from the things that come out of our mouths.

This week I challenge you to consider what is coming out of your mouth.

In the days when I was overly focused on my food intake, I wrote down everything that I ate.

What if every word that we said was written down? Would we be pleased? Would we want others to read it?

I know I need to do some work in that area.

## Action Step

Practice pausing this week. Pause before eating. Pause before speaking.

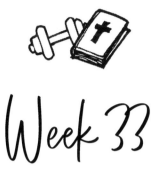

# Week 33

*I will hear what God the Lord will speak, for He will speak peace to His people and to His saints; but let them not turn back to folly.*

**Psalm 85:8 (NKJV)**

Comparison. It is a trap we all fall into at one time or another. Unfortunately, comparison has no boundaries. It hits women of all ages and in all stages of life.

But we can choose to identify it and change it.

*I will hear what God the Lord will speak.*

Will I?

Will I choose to hear what He says about me in His Word rather than what social media tells me I should be?

Will I choose to listen to His voice rather than the ones in my head telling me I am not enough?

Will I let His Spirit guide me when making decisions rather than copy the way someone else is doing it?

God speaks. He speaks through His Word, His Spirit, our sisters and brothers in Christ.

Comparison makes us anxious. It makes us feel less than or superior to. It gives rise to competition.

God's Word brings peace — peace in our hearts and peace in our relationships.

Will you listen to Him speak to you this week?

Are you feeling the weight of comparison in your life? Dig into God's Word and let His peace fill you this week. And do not turn back.

> **Action Step**
>
> Make a list of what makes you unique. Thank God for making you a special and loved person.

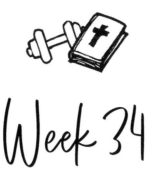

# Week 34

*Happy are all who search for God and always do his will, rejecting compromise with evil and walking only in his paths.*

**Psalm 119:2-3 (TLB)**

Seeking God, obeying His commands, and doing His will bring happiness.

We can apply this to our healthy living journey.

Living fit and free means we are seeking God's will about how to care for our unique bodies and not compromising with diets, gimmicks, and quick fixes.

I have learned that the most important part of my healthy life is keeping my eyes on Jesus and following His path for me. When I get distracted with feelings of insecurity or when comparison rears its ugly head, I am not happy. When I start searching for quick fixes online or start reading someone's social media transformation post, I am not happy. But when I go back to seeking to do His will in this area of my life and searching His Word for the truth it says about me, I have peace and happiness in my life.

Are you following a healthy living journey that makes you happy?

Are you happy with the approach you have chosen to care for your one special body that God has entrusted to you?

I hope you are.

You are more than halfway through this book. Are you finding true happiness in following Jesus and His unique path for you?

I cried too many tears over a number on a scale and wasted a lot of time being unhappy in my life because I was not walking God's path for me in this area of my life.

If you find yourself in a similar predicament, spend time in prayer this week. Seek God. And obey Him when He responds. I know that He will. And once you choose to walk His path, you will start feeling better.

> ## Action Step
>
> Take a walk outside every day this week.

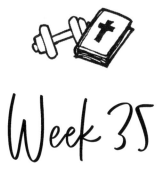

# Week 35

*We demolish arguments and every pretension that sets itself up against the knowledge of God, and we take captive every thought to make it obedient to Christ.*

## 2 Corinthians 10:5 (NIV)

Do you ever stop to think about what you are thinking about? Just like the television or the radio that is playing in the background, so are your thoughts.

We might not always be aware of exactly what is on the station, but something is playing, and every now and then we pick up a few words.

Consider the following scenarios:

A girl whose father left the family when she was young. Does that mean all men will leave her? The teen who did not have a date for prom. Will she always be alone? What's wrong with me that I can't get a date? What about the one who was picked last for the team in gym class? (Right here!) Does that mean I will get overlooked for the job opening? You want to start running, but someone once told you you're not a runner. You want to set a goal, but someone once said you never follow through with anything.

And then there are words that are *meant* to hurt.

People can be uncaring and downright mean. Even though their words were not true, they stuck. We might not think of them every day, but when something comes up, they are there. The point is this: We must recognize the thoughts and the tapes that play in our heads. Consider the thoughts that come floating by - the ones you entertain. What experiences have you bookmarked that you may not even realize until something comes up, and then you are right back in that moment? It is time to take those thoughts captive and replace them with new tapes.

Recognize those words and experiences for what they are. Cassette tapes and 8-tracks (I am totally dating myself here!) are antiques now and nearly non-existent. So why do we let those tapes in our heads keep playing? They are out of date. They no longer exist.

When those thoughts come up and those tapes start playing, switch the station. Turn to God's Word and focus on His truth.

## Action Step

Journal every day this week. Write down your thoughts. What are you thinking? Do you need to replace some negative thoughts with positive ones?

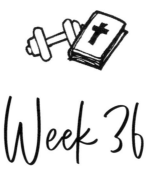

# Week 36

*Yet in all these things we are more than conquerors and gain an overwhelming victory through Him who loved us [so much that He died for us].*

**Romans 8:37 (AMP)**

Who doesn't like to win?

We all want to be successful in our endeavors. If we play a game, we want to win. If we enter a challenge, we want to meet the challenge. If we set a goal, we want to complete it successfully. And if we are cheering for a team, we want our team to win.

People do not set goals or make resolutions so they can fail. Teams do not go into games planning to lose. We all want to be victorious.

In Christ, we can be!

Now, I am not saying that a prayer will get you or your team a win.

What I am saying is that in life, in our personal lives, when we commit our ways to Christ and trust and obey, He will help us be victorious.

I believe we can be victorious on our health and fitness journey when we seek Christ and allow Him to change us from the inside out.

He can help us conquer the cravings and the negative self-talk that often holds us back, and by His Spirit, we can embrace new mercies each day as we work to make positive changes in our lives.

Do you feel as if you are fighting a losing battle in some area of your life? Take some time to submit it to the Lord. Ask Him for help. Ask Him to help you with a game plan. Then obey His Word and follow His lead.

May this be the year that you are victorious!

## Action Step

Play a game this week. Sign up for a race. Try a new sport.

Week 36

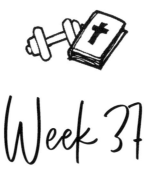

# Week 37

*Before I formed you in the womb I knew you; before you were born I sanctified you; I ordained you a prophet to the nations.*

**Jeremiah 1:5 (NKJV)**

Just as these words came to Jeremiah, let them wash over you this week.

Before He formed you, He knew you. He loved you.

If you are a parent, especially a mother, you know the impact of these words. That child you prayed for, longed for, and then carried in your womb, you loved that child before he or she was ever born.

So it is with you and the Heavenly Father. He has always loved you. *And* He has set you apart. He has plans for you. No matter your age or stage of life, God has a plan. It is not too late to accomplish that purpose He has for your life.

The reason I help women develop a healthy life that is sustainable is *so that* they can do all that God has created them to do.

It is *so that* you can love and serve those around you.

The focus on living a fit and healthy life is to *free* us up to be the best version of ourselves, not for a transformation picture or a bikini body, but to share with the world that unique thing God has entrusted you with, whether it is in a small corner or on a big stage.

God loves you, dear one, and He has created you for a specific purpose. Start living it out today.

### Action Step

Look at baby pictures, your own or those belonging to members of your family, and feel God's love for you.

# Week 38

*Then the Lord said to Moses, "Come up to Me on the mountain and be there; and I will give you tablets of stone, and the law and commandments which I have written, that you may teach them."*

**Exodus 24:12 (NKJV)**

Be there.

God invited Moses to meet with Him and simply asked Him to be there.

How often do you approach your daily prayers by giving God a list of wants and needs and then rushing off to get on with your day?

God had something for Moses. He had something for Moses to share with others.

But first God asked Moses to be there.

I wonder if you or I have missed out on something because we skipped that most important step.

Am I asking for things but not stopping long enough for God to give me what I need?

This reminds me of my word of the year a few years ago: Breathe.

I had to learn the importance of pausing — pausing to be with the One who has all that you and I need.

When you spend time with the Lord, are you really there?

Do you have difficulty being present in the moment? With the Lord? With your children? With your spouse? With that friend who needs to talk?

We live in a fast-paced world, but we do not have to get caught up in the fast lane.

God has what you need. He is just asking that you come to Him and be there so He can give it to you.

Will you take some time to be with Jesus this week?

## Action Step

Prioritize alone time with Jesus this week. Spend uninterrupted time with someone special.

Week 38

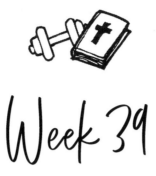

# Week 39

*A heart at peace gives life to the body, but envy rots the bones.*

**Proverbs 14:30 (NIV)**

"All of God's girls have issues." This is a quote from Lysa TerKeurst in her book *Made to Crave*. This statement has stuck with me since I first read the book over eight years ago.

We do not always know what is going on in a person's heart or behind closed doors and off the grid of social media.

Even the person who looks all put together on the outside — family, career, body, you name it — has issues. There is a struggle, a fear, a regret, an insecurity, something that she is dealing with and you don't see it.

When we compare our lives with others based on what we

see, we are not seeing the whole picture. When we desire to be more like so-and-so, or have X, Y, or Z like another person, we do not know what else is going on.

There is good and bad in every situation. There are ups and downs and highs and lows.

When we desire someone else's life, we must remember that the good we see also includes some not-so-good.

God has entrusted you with this life, this body, this reality.

*Entrusted* it to you. This is the life He knows is right for you.

I don't know about you, but I think I will choose peace and the life God knows I can handle.

How about you?

## Action Step

Look for someone to encourage this week. Send a note. Schedule a coffee date. Invite someone to join you for a walk.

# Week 40

*For you were once darkness, but now you are light in the Lord. Walk as children of light (for the fruit of the Spirit is in all goodness, righteousness, and truth), finding out what is acceptable to the Lord.*

### Ephesians 5:8-10 (NKJV)

Walk in the light you now know.

Throughout our lives, God peels back layers. He takes us one step at a time to reveal more of His plan. He takes us step by step, illuminating our paths in stages as we are prepared to see it and to follow.

When I began sharing my faith and fitness journey, I was a Beachbody coach. It was what I knew at the time and the avenue that allowed me to share my story. Eventually, I realized that I did not want to be tied to a product, nor did I have to be, to help women break free from dieting and discover how to feel good in their bodies now.

God is shining a light for us, revealing what is acceptable to Him in our everyday lives. To know Jesus is the ultimate of going from darkness to light. But that is simply the first step to walking in the light.

On our journey, we must remain open to His goodness, righteousness, and truth. For each of us, it is different and unique. He has a specific plan designed for you and one designed for me.

I followed that light originally to become a coach, but then He provided light in a different direction, and I had to follow, not only for my business approach but also for my healthy living approach.

Are you walking in the light? Has He changed the direction of the light? Have you followed?

To walk as a child of the light means you are moving forward, taking action.

How is your progress?

He wants you to remain in the light — in *His* light — so that He can guide you where you can become the best version of yourself.

Be open to what He wants to reveal next.

## Action Step

Take an early morning or late evening walk that requires a light. Think about walking as a child of the light.

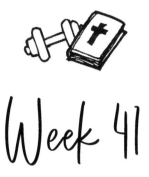

# Week 41

*Let the words of my mouth and the meditation of my heart be acceptable in Your sight, O Lord, my strength and my Redeemer.*

**Psalm 19:14 (NKJV)**

Our words and our thoughts, they are everything. What is going on in our minds eventually comes out of our mouths in words spoken to ourselves and to others.

This week, let's focus on our thoughts and words about ourselves. How we think about and speak to ourselves impacts how we show up for ourselves and how we interact with others.

The Lord knows all things. He knows your thoughts, and He hears your words.

Certainly all kinds of thoughts come to our minds.

Have you ever had a thought and wondered where that even came from?

Thoughts are darting around in our minds all the time. But where do you pause, and which of those thoughts do you entertain?

Meditations are those thoughts to which we give extended time. They are the thoughts that we engage with and think on over and over again.

What we think about most frequently becomes our topics of conversation.

Much of my life I spent worrying about my weight. I worried about gaining weight. I worried about how people saw me and if they judged my body size. I thought about ways to lose weight and how I failed at being able to look a certain way.

Those thoughts came out in the way I spoke to myself, thus feeding my insecurities and preventing me from engaging with other people. When I would get together with a friend, our conversations would turn to our "weight problems," and we would leave that interaction feeling worse than when we met up. All the while, those words and thoughts were not acceptable to the Lord.

He created me. He created you. He is pleased with His creation.

When I began to change my thoughts, my conversations changed, as did my confidence in who I was and how I was created.

Our verse this week is simple, yet it can change everything.

When you notice thoughts that are not helpful or when you

hear yourself speaking things about yourself that are defeating, speak this verse out loud.

> ## Action Step
> Make this verse a daily prayer this week, starting today.

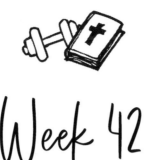

# Week 42

*Rest in the Lord, and wait patiently for Him; do not fret because of him who prospers in his way, because of the man who brings wicked schemes to pass. Cease from anger, and forsake wrath; do not fret — it only causes harm.*

### Psalm 37:7-8 (NKJV)

Rest. I am not good with it. I rarely take days off from working out.

Yes, I get seven or eight hours of sleep a night, but I am up and at it early and don't allow myself much time throughout the day when I am not doing something — working, cleaning, exercising, etc. I am often doing something *I think* is productive.

But rest.

Rest *is* productive. It is necessary. God created a weekly Sabbath for rest. He commands us to honor the Sabbath.

This is something I am working on. Do you struggle with rest as well?

These verses in Psalms say, "rest in the Lord and wait patiently for Him...do not fret."

He is always at work so you and I do not have to be.

Yes, we need to be obedient to do what He has called us to do, but part of that obedience is resting.

Rest in Him.

I am going to practice resting a little more today, and I am going to commit to more rest. That is not being lazy when it is resting in Him. It is being obedient.

How are you going to practice resting this week? If you do not know where to start, try sitting quietly, taking a break from social media, or taking a leisurely walk.

## Action Step

Create time for the Sabbath this week. It does not have to be on Sunday, but take a time-out.

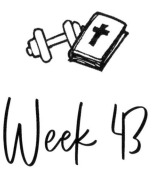

# Week 43

*For Scripture says to Pharaoh: "I raised you up for this very purpose, that I might display my power in you and that my name might be proclaimed in all the earth."*

**Romans 9:17 (NIV)**

God had a specific purpose and plan in mind when He created you. Whatever is happening in your life right now has meaning.

This verse in Romans is actually taken from God's word to Pharaoh through Moses in the book of Exodus. Among the plagues and all that was going on, God was in control.

God has a plan and a purpose for all that He allows to happen. The end result, the purpose, is for God to be lifted up.

Your purpose in life is not to lose five pounds or achieve a certain finish time at your next race or even to raise a child who will be the President of the United States or the Pope.

Your purpose in life is to allow God to have His way in and through you. It is to allow Him to show up in your life and be glorified. We are here to point others to Jesus.

What we are going through brings us into closer relationships to Him and allows His power to be seen in our lives.

If you are wondering what your purpose is or what God's plan is for you in this season, know that it is all for His glory.

Know that He loves you so much that He wants you to be part of His big plan.

I have allowed trivial things to sidetrack me from His power and His presence in my life. They have distracted me from what He is wanting to do in me and through me.

When you and I do that, we miss a chance to be closer to Him. We miss the chance to see Him work in the lives of those around us.

Will you, with me, surrender to His plan and purpose for you this week?

He is God, and His way is good.

## Action Step

Look for opportunities to serve others this week.

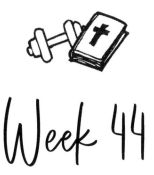

# Week 44

*If you find honey, eat just enough — too much of it, and you will vomit.*

**Proverbs 25:16 (NIV)**

It is a relatively simple concept — eat just enough, otherwise you will make yourself sick if you stuff yourself.

Too often we dismiss seemingly trivial topics and assume they are not important to the Lord.

How many times have you heard someone say (perhaps you have said it to yourself), "God has more important things to deal with than _____"?

We tend to take the big things to God or consult His Word on major decisions, but the little things, well, we try to navigate those on our own. Or we discuss those issues with a friend and look for answers on the internet.

But the truth is everything is important to the Lord.

We can find guidance in His Word for every issue that comes up in our lives.

Take this simple verse found in Proverbs: "If you find honey, eat just enough — too much of it, and you will vomit."

This is a perfect place to start your healthy living plan, or the upcoming holiday season (if you have been reading this book since January).

Eat enough to satisfy but not so much that you are stuffed and feeling sick afterwards.

I imagine most of us have experienced a time when we have eaten until we were uncomfortable.

Take the holidays. How many times will you hear, "Ugh, I ate too much"?

Many holidays include sweets and treats and excessive amounts of food. There is nothing wrong with sweets and treats and holiday food. But in excess, nothing good comes from those things. When we consume these things in excess, they are no longer enjoyable. We end up feeling miserable instead.

The next time you are faced with an abundance of food choices, eat just enough. Enjoy the goodies. Let the kiddos enjoy them as well. But also enjoy the time with family and friends. Get outside and get some fresh air.

Let this be your motto for a happy, healthy holiday season!

## Action Step

Spend extra time outside this week. Take a short walk. Don't forget to bundle up if it's chilly. Fresh air is so refreshing for your mind and your body.

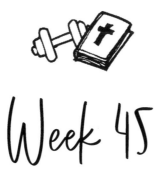

# Week 45

*Remember the former things of old, for I am God, and there is no other; I am God, and there is none like Me.*

**Isaiah 46:9 (NKJV)**

"Remember the former things of old…"

Wait a minute. A few chapters earlier we were being told to "remember not." Now we're supposed to remember?

There is a time for remembering and a time for letting go.

For this week, let's focus on this verse and do what it says: Remember.

It is good to remember God's work in our lives. We need to take time to reflect on what He has done, where we have come from, and how He took us from one place to the next.

When we reflect, we are reminded of the goodness of God. Looking back helps us see the blessings we have experienced along the way. We can also look back on our old self and call to mind the changes that have taken place.

When I look back, I see the desert that He brought me out of and how He used that experience in my life to grow me so I can help women now.

During difficult times, I am reminded how God has always come through and has never left me alone. I can be confident He will do that again.

When you take a moment to remember, what do you recall?

Do you keep a journal? What about photos?

Although God is present and working in our lives all the time, sometimes glancing back through a journal or photos will jog your memory of various times, seasons, and situations when God did something truly amazing.

There is no God like our God. Spend some time reflecting on how He has shown up in your life. Expect Him to continue to show up.

## Action Step

Take a look back. You are nearing the end of this journey. What improvements have you made? What has changed? How will you continue on this path?

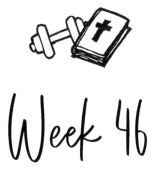

# Week 46

*Let everything that has breath praise the Lord.*

**Psalm 150:6a (NKJV)**

It seems so simple, yet do we praise God? How often do you praise Him?

Do you praise Him for the breath in your lungs?

Breathing is something that we do not even think about. We don't have to, yet when the breathing stops, that's it.

We have been talking about health and wellness, but the emphasis is on faith and how it all ties together.

Looking at this scripture and thinking about breathing makes me think about working out and exercising. We are so much more aware of our breath when we are working out.

And so I wonder if we can tie this together?

As we are moving and exercising, could it become an act of worship? Could it cause your thoughts to go to how you are blessed with the privilege to move, blessed with the privilege simply to inhale and exhale?

This week I challenge you to look at your workout a bit differently. With each breath, will you praise Him?

> **Action Step**
>
> Start a gratitude journal. Establish a daily gratitude practice that you will continue beyond this devotional.

Week 46

# Week 47

*When Jesus saw her, he called her forward and said to her, "Woman, you are set free from your infirmity." Then he put his hands on her, and immediately she straightened up and praised God.*

### Luke 13:12-13 (NIV)

This woman was set free by the power of Christ *to glorify God*.

When God does a work in our lives, it is for a purpose.

While I struggled with body image, I believed that my life's mission was to lose weight. But on a deeper level, I simply wanted to be free.

I wanted to be free of the inner turmoil this struggle caused. I wanted to be free from daily worries about how I looked and what other people thought of me. I wanted to be free from being driven by numbers on a scale.

God did set me free. But He did not set me free simply to make my life easier. He set me free *so that* I could glorify Him with this story. He set me free *so that* I could share with others that He can set them free too.

When you are overcome with a struggle — whether it is an illness, a financial or a relational problem, or any weight or worry — and then you are set free, you want to let others know. You want them to know there is a better way.

I know what it's like to live based on numbers.

I know what it's like to worry constantly about what others think of me.

I know what it's like to feel lonely even when you're not alone.

I know what it's like to be anxious all of the time.

Once I was free from those things, I wanted to share it.

When people asked me how I let those things go, I wanted to tell them that it was by God's grace.

What has God done in your life?

He did it for a purpose.

Are you sharing it? Are you praising Him for it? Are you giving Him glory?

He has done something *in* you so He can do something *through* you.

> ## Action Step
>
> Share with someone what God has done for you. Tell them about the changes He has made in you on this journey.

# Week 48

*Then Moses said to the Lord, "O my Lord, I am not eloquent, neither before nor since You have spoken to Your servant; but I am slow of speech and slow of tongue."*

**Exodus 4:10 (NKJV)**

Have you ever felt like you were not enough?

Not smart enough.

Not pretty enough.

Not successful enough.

Not thin enough.

Not good enough.

Not enough for my spouse.

Not enough for my kids.

Not enough for my friends.

Moses, one of the heroes of the Old Testament, felt like he was not enough.

And truthfully, he was not enough.

In fact, you and I are not enough.

*But God.*

With God, Moses was enough.

With God, you are enough.

With God, I am enough.

God made Moses enough in spite of his weaknesses.

God makes you enough regardless of your struggles.

He makes me enough even though I fail.

Who says you are not enough? God does not.

He picked you and said, *"I will make you enough."*

## Action Step

Remind yourself daily this week that you are enough — with God.

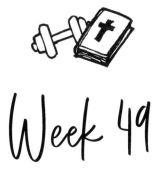

# Week 49

*In the morning, Lord, you hear my voice; in the morning I lay my requests before you and wait expectantly.*

**Psalm 5:3 (NIV)**

Mornings matter.

Whether you are a morning person or not, it is imperative to start your day with the Lord if you want to head in the right direction.

You've likely been developing this habit over the last several weeks.

This does not mean that you must make your morning prayers into a long and lengthy experience. It can be as simple as reciting a verse like "This is the day the Lord has made; I will rejoice and be glad in it." Or praying, "Lord, I give this day to You. Please lead me and guide me and help me to keep my eyes on You."

My Faith and Fitness Framework™ is about building a healthy life on a foundation of faith.

Everything starts with Jesus — a new project, a big goal, a new day, a healthy living plan.

Invite Him to lead and guide you and to be part of your day.

If you prefer doing your devotions or Bible study in the afternoon or before bed, that is perfect. But I still encourage you to meet Him each morning, even if for a few moments. He is there to hear your words and to respond to your requests.

Now it is time to watch for Him to show up in your day. I know He will!

> **Action Step**
>
> Set your alarm every morning this week with enough time to meet with the Lord in the morning.

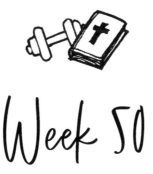

# Week 50

*So do not throw away your confidence; it will be richly rewarded.*

**Hebrews 10:35 (NIV)**

Low self-confidence. That was one of my attributes growing up. Lacking confidence or self-esteem. Worried about what others thought of me. Not sure of myself or my opinions.

But I had it a bit wrong. Yes, I struggled with all things having to do with myself, but do you notice a theme in this?

Self.

To be sure, we should feel good in our skin. We need to be bold and confident. I want my boys to be strong men and feel good about themselves.

But the thing with confidence is this: It is not really about self; it is about who lives in us.

Your faith, your hope, your confidence should be placed in Christ.

We are to live confidently. We are to walk our lives with confidence. But the confidence comes from knowing Jesus, relying on Him, and trusting in Him.

This passage of scripture is talking about living a life of faith and reliance on God. It is about having the hope of eternity and a confidence in what is to come. It is about having the confidence that He paid the price for our sin and for us to live in eternity with Him.

I had low self-confidence because I was putting my confidence in myself. I based it on how I felt about my reflection in the mirror and my abilities or lack thereof. It was misguided and misdirected.

Your confidence needs to be in Jesus. When you look to Him, you can be secure in His love for you and His plan for you – both today and in the future.

May you walk confidently knowing that in Christ all things are good and His plan for you is good.

## Action Step

God has done some amazing things in your life over the last several weeks. Be confident in what He has done. This week, notice how you are carrying yourself differently. Notice the smile that comes more easily. Stand tall. Thank God for what He has done and ask Him to continue this work.

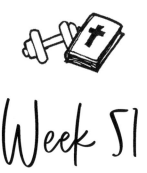

# Week 51

*When Peter saw him, he asked, "Lord, what about him?" Jesus answered, "If I want him to remain alive until I return, what is that to you? You must follow me."*

### John 21:21-22 (NIV)

Have you had this same thought?

Perhaps you have looked at someone else's life and wondered why they have it all together or do not have your same struggles, difficulties, challenges, trials.

I've done it.

When I did not like myself or my body, I wondered why she didn't have those same insecure feelings.

When I was single and then when my first marriage ended, I

was sure I would be alone for the rest of my life. I looked at others and wanted to know why they had all the friends and found the perfect man.

God, why can't You do that for me?

God, don't You love me like You love her?

God, why is my life crumbling around me while she's getting the guy, losing the weight, building a successful business, becoming a best-selling author, etc.?

Sometimes we get so distracted by everything going on around us that we miss the wonderful works God is doing *in* us and *for* us. If we would only pause for a moment, we would see that He always has our best interest in mind. He is a loving Father who has the perfect plan for our individual lives.

How God works in someone else does not take away from what He is doing in your life. God knows the whole story and sees the entire picture.

How He chooses to bless another does not add to or take away from anything He can and will and wants to do in your life. We must simply follow Him. Because following Him, running the race He has marked out for you, is the best place to be.

This week, He is telling you not to worry about someone else's life but only to make sure you are following Him. He will take care of the rest.

## Action Step

If you are going to continue living differently, you must keep your eyes on your own paper. This is about you, not about what someone else is doing or what is happening in another's life. Are there social media accounts you need to unsubscribe from or habits you need to change to avoid comparing yourself to others?

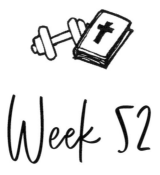

# Week 52

*My flesh and my heart may fail, but God is the strength of my heart and my portion forever.*

### Psalm 73:26 (NIV)

I fell off the wagon.

I will start over on Monday.

I really messed up this time.

I am never going to get it right.

Have you ever said any of those things? Maybe something close to it?

Have you ever felt like a failure — as a parent, as a spouse, on a project, on your healthy living journey? I have — in all of those areas. And more than once!

We are going to mess up. We will get it wrong.

Part of any process — how to parent, how to become a better spouse, how to live a healthy life — includes some bumps in the road.

"My flesh and my heart may fail, but God is the strength of my heart and my portion forever."

But God.

Because of God's strength, we can try again. Because He gives us all that we need, we can get back at it and keep on going.

On our own, we will fail. Even with God, we will struggle. But He will be there with strength and with all we need to move forward on the path that He is leading.

I am not sure in which area of your life you feel like you have messed up, but I know that God has what you need to refocus.

Psalm 73:28 (NKJV) says, "But it is good for me to draw near to God; I have put my trust in the Lord."

Dear friend, draw near to God this week. Let Him be your strength and give you all that you need to face your struggle. He is trustworthy.

## Action Step

Progress over perfection. Your life, including this healthy living journey, never will be perfect. Be okay with slow and steady progress. There might even be pauses along the way. That's okay.

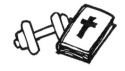

# Final Day

*For if you remain completely silent at this time, relief and deliverance will arise for the Jews from another place, but you and your father's house will perish. Yet who knows whether you have come to the kingdom for such a time as this?*

**Esther 4:14 (NKJV)**

I don't know about you, but I have always stumbled over the first part of this verse and focused on the last sentence, a question actually.

Recently I paused and read the entire verse. God had a plan, and it *would be* executed.

It was not a question of whether or not the Jews would be delivered. The question was would Esther participate in God's plan?

His plan was going to be executed back in Esther's day, and

it will be executed today. The question is whether you will participate in it.

God invites us to be part of His plan. He did not need Esther, and He does not need you or me. But He invites us into the story.

Instead of looking around and pointing to someone else, or sitting back and letting someone else go, stand up. Raise your hand and let God know you are ready. Tell Him you want to get involved.

God created you and placed you on this earth at this time for a reason. Step fully and confidently into your life and your calling.

You have come to this point in your life for such a time as this.

## Final Words

God has a plan and a purpose for you, and it is so much more than weight loss. The reason you are pursuing a fit life is for freedom. It is *so that* you can do what God has called you to do.

Here's to living fit *and* free!

Final Day **211**

# Epilogue

Thank you for picking up this devotional. Whether you have taken an entire year or a few weeks to reach this page, there is a reason you have this book in hand. No matter your age or stage of life, God has a purpose for you. And He wants you to know that you are not alone.

I would love to connect with you. If you're still reading this book, I want to travel this journey with you. If you are finished and wondering what's next, I would love to help you keep going.

Some ways we can connect:

Faith and Fitness Sisterhood, my free Facebook group — facebook.com/groups/1413320032061119/

Faith and Fitness Membership Community — marshaapsley.com/community

Visit my website, marshaapsley.com

Email me — marsha@marshaapsley.com

More by Marsha Apsley (found on Amazon)

*40 Days of Faith and Fitness*
*40 Days of Faith and Fitness for Tweens and Teens*
*Turn Your Holidays into Holy-Days*
*Faith and Fitness Study Guide*

# About the Author

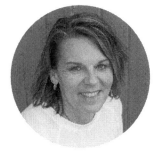

Marsha Apsley desires to live according to 1 Corinthians 10:31, "So whether you eat or drink or whatever you do, do it all for the glory of God." She believes that God wants to be part of our everyday lives including how we eat and drink and how we view our reflection in the mirror. She cried far too many tears over a number on a scale but is thankful that God can now use those experiences to help other women find the freedom they're looking for.

Marsha's first devotional was *40 Days of Faith and Fitness: A Devotional Journal*. Since then, she has written *Turn Your Holidays into Holy-Days: 31-Day Guide to a Happy, Healthy December* as well as a tweens and teens version of *40 Days of Faith and Fitness*.

She is a counselor and is passionate about helping women live fit and free. She does this by teaching her Faith and Fitness Framework™ and providing support and accountability in her Faith and Fitness Membership Community. It is important for women to focus on whole-person health and wellness with an inside out approach. She believes that a healthy lifestyle needs to be built on a firm foundation of faith.

Marsha Apsley is a wife and mom of two sons. She loves to run and bike and believes every day is better with chocolate and coffee. For more support and encouragement on your faith and fitness journey, please visit her website at www.marshaapsley.com or find her on social media, @marshaapsley.

Made in the USA
Las Vegas, NV
12 March 2022